Foreword

Barts and The London have an illustrious history. Barts is the oldest hospital in Britain (formed in 1123) and The London Hospital Medical College was the first medical school given a charter for medical education (in 1785). The schools of the two hospitals merged in 1995 to form Barts and The London School of Medicine and Dentistry. Many distinguished physicians and eminent scientists worked at Barts and The London and, in spite of their fame, medical students have, in the course of my teaching at Barts and the London, revealed that they did not know who are the people whose names are on the walls of the school's Institutes, buildings and lecture rooms. For example the Garrod Building which accommodates the school offices is well known among the students but not who Garrod was or what he achieved.

The individuals recognised through their names on our walls have made valuable contributions to science, medicine and teaching. This prompted the idea for a collection of brief histories of the people named on the walls of the school that would be of interest to students thinking of joining Barts and The London, students already here, and even the wider public. This booklet relates only to the names of individuals named on the walls of the medical sections of the school and does not extend to dentistry and the two parent hospitals.

I discussed the idea with Dr Alan Bailey FRCP, an alumnus of Barts. He kindly agreed to take on the task. This booklet is the result. It gives a brief account of individuals who have literally made their mark at Barts and The London. Their names are part of the fabric of the Medical School.

Sir Nicholas Wald FRS FRCP
Wolfson Institute of Preventive Medi
Barts and The London School of Mec
December 2015

Published by

Wolfson Institute of Preventive Medicine
Charterhouse Square, London EC1M 6BQ, UK

British Library Cataloguing in Publication Data
A catalogue record for this book is available from the British Library

Distribution:
Wolfson Institute of Preventive Medicine
Barts and The London School of Medicine and Dentistry
Charterhouse Square, London EC1M 6BQ, UK
Tel: +44 (0)20 7882 3850
Fax: +44 (0)20 7882 6270
E-mail: wolfson@qmul.ac.uk

ISBN 978-1-898227-02-1

Printed and bound by

The Copy Shop Queen Mary University of London

The printing of this booklet was funded by Barts Charity

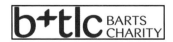

Acknowledgements

Many people have helped in gathering the information in this booklet and I thank them all. In particular I would like to thank Louise Schweitzer for her edits on the text, the Medical Illustration Department of Barts and The London NHS Trust for provision of photographs, and Michelle Beegan, Dallas Allen and Mia Kalezic for putting together the final version.

Alan Bailey
January 2016

The Institutes/buildings/rooms and their locations

Name	Location
Abernethy Building	Whitechapel
Bainbridge Room	West Smithfield
Blizard Building	Whitechapel
Boyle Room	West Smithfield
Robin Brook Centre	West Smithfield
Yvonne Carter Building	Whitechapel
Clark-Kennedy Lecture Theatre	Whitechapel
Sir Anthony Dawson Hall	Charterhouse Square
Doniach Gallery	Whitechapel
John Langdon Down House	Charterhouse Square
Floyer House	Whitechapel
Garrod Building	Whitechapel
William Harvey Research Institute	Charterhouse Square
Michael Mason Room	Whitechapel
Perrin Lecture Theatre	Whitechapel
Dean Rees House	Charterhouse Square
Paterson Ross Lecture Theatre	West Smithfield
Joseph Rotblat Building	Charterhouse Square
Thompson-Yates Room	Whitechapel
Turnbull Centre	Mile End
Sir John Vane Science Centre	Charterhouse Square
Derek Willoughby Lecture Theatre	Charterhouse Square
Wingate Institute	Whitechapel
Wolfson Institute of Preventive Medicine	Charterhouse Square

Table of contents

John Abernethy
1764 - 1831

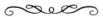

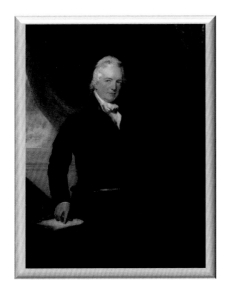

John Abernethy founded the present tradition of medical education at Barts Hospital. Not only was he one of the earliest surgeon-teachers, he was also a practical fund-raiser and political activist who persuaded the hospital governors to spend money on vital facilities needed to train new surgeons and maintain the reputation of the hospital. His lectures, advertised in *The Times* and initially held in the Abernethy house at Bartholomew Close, inspired and impressed students with a new zest for their profession and it was fitting that he was selected to inaugurate the new Barts Lecture Theatre on October 1ˢᵗ, 1822, before an audience of 406 people. Progressively, he encouraged medical experiments alongside surgical practice, a tradition which continues to this day.

Abernethy studied surgery under William Blizard at the London Hospital, Percivall Pott of Barts and John Hunter at St. George's Hospital. He was appointed Assistant Surgeon to Barts in 1787 and Surgeon in 1815, but he remained a Lecturer. In 1795, he created the Medical and Philosophical Society, members of which were responsible for starting the Library. In 1828, he donated his collection of surgical specimens to a collection which grew to become the Pathology Museum.

In John Thornton's biography, Abernethy is painted as a slightly churlish eccentric. Leaving his house one day, he kicked his foot against a paving stone where the road was under repair. He shouted to a workman to remove it. 'And where shall I take it?' asked the workman. 'Take it to Hell for all I care' came the reply. 'Maybe' said the Irishman, 'if I take it to Heaven, it will be more out of Your Honour's way.'

He is also known for his medical writings. Carefully observed case histories describe patients with head injuries who were admitted to Barts, purged, bled and amazingly recovered! Another series examined the ill-effects of venesection. Despite this common practice in the eighteenth century, Abernethy recognised that the inflammation which may arise around the site was probably due to ....*the lancet which was employed which was envenomously affected whereby the absorption of virulent matter produced the inflammation.* More writing describes experiments on tadpoles and rabbits, presumably easily obtained in his garden, if sometimes neglected when he travelled away from London.

In 1796, John Abernethy was elected Fellow of the Royal Society, and in 1826 President of the Royal College of Surgeons. He was a founding member and early President of the Royal Medical Chirurgical Society, which became the Royal Society of Medicine. Many of his proposals were incorporated in various Medical Acts of the late 18th century.

John Abernethy suffered progressive ill health and, aged sixty five, he retired increasingly to his country house in Enfield. When he died there on April 20th, 1831, Barts had become the largest medical school in London.

The Abernethy Building is on the Whitechapel campus.

Francis Arthur Bainbridge
1874-1921

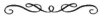

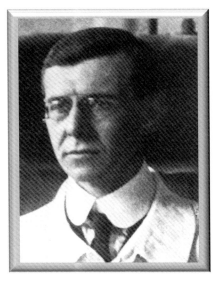

Francis Bainbridge made a vital contribution to understanding the physiology of exercise. He was able to prove that an increase of pressure on the venous side of the heart resulted in an increased pulse rate, partly due to inhibition of the vagal tone, and partly by reflex excitation of the accelerator mechanism. This was the exact reverse of earlier theories enshrined in Marey's Law – that rising ventricular pressure slowed heart rate. His text books *Essentials of Physiology*, 1914, written with Professor Menzies from Newcastle and *Physiology of Muscular Exercise,* 1919, proved very popular with students and remain in print to this day. Not only did they demonstrate a physiological breakthrough, but they also coalesced a vast amount of previously disconnected material into a concise and coherent thesis.

Francis Bainbridge was born in Stockton-on-Tees in 1874 and won a scholarship to The Leys School, Cambridge. He went up to Trinity College, achieving a First Class Honours Degree in Natural Sciences in 1897. An appointment as Junior Demonstrator in Physiology at Barts in 1900 was followed by an MB, Cambridge and MRCP, London, with an election as FRCP in 1909. He also held appointments at Great Ormond Street and carried out research in the physiology department of University College.

Bainbridge was a competent bacteriologist whose work on the influence of proteins on bacteria and on the classification of the paratyphoid bacteria became the subject of the Milroy Lecture at the Royal College of Physicians in 1912. But his primary interest remained physiology and, when he became Professor of Physiology at the Newcastle School of Medicine at Durham University in 1911, he was able to continue the research into kidney function which he had begun at Guys Hospital in London.

The outbreak of World War One was responsible for his transfer to a military hospital in Newcastle. One year later in 1915, his skills were required at Barts when he was appointed Professor of Physiology, for active research into the effects of poisonous gases. Francis Bainbridge was also involved in educating civilian and military personnel in the defences required against such intangible weaponry. He remained at Barts for the remainder of his working life.

He was an enthusiastic researcher, never happier than when trying to perform a difficult procedure on an animal. Posterity holds differing views on his appeal as a lecturer; some accounts describe him as short and unimpressive, whilst others believed him to be an excellent expounder of his subject. But if his pupils varied in admiration, medical collaborators were united in enjoying a lifelong scholarship with him. Bainbridge worked with many great names in physiology including Henry Dale (similarly from Leys and Trinity, Cambridge) and C.L. Evans of University College. Their experiments using their heart, lung and kidney preparation, and published in the *Journal of Physiology*, 1921, are still occasionally in use today.

Francis Bainbridge suffered intermittent ill health in his later years and died in 1921.

The Bainbridge Room is on the West Smithfield campus

Sir William Blizard
1743 - 1835

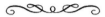

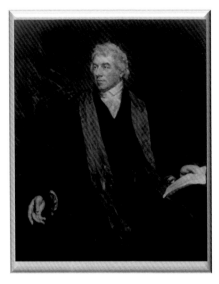

William Blizard founded the London Hospital Medical College in 1785, the first medical school in the capital. His pioneering career in medicine and social work reflected a wide range of skills and interests from surgery to public welfare, volunteer soldiering, law and order and even the writing of poetry. He was elected Fellow of the Royal Society in 1787, knighted in 1803 and continued operating until he was 84. He was twice the senior Surgeon of the Royal College of Surgeons, Master, 1814, and President, 1822.

Blizard was born at Barn Elms in Surrey, the son of a local auctioneer. He became apprenticed to a surgeon in Mortlake before attending lectures by Percivall Pott at St. Bartholomew's and studied surgery at the London Hospital where he was appointed Surgeon in 1780. As a member of the Honourable Artillery Company (HAC), Blizard became involved in their City division, formed after the successful quelling of the Gordon Riots in 1780. He often accompanied the HAC on city sorties, writing frequent letters to the authorities with ideas for reducing crime and violence in the late 1700s, before Robert Peel's early policemen, 'Peelers' were launched in 1820.

Blizard's initiatives included encouraging local industries to employ poor people; keeping sick and malnourished patients at his hospital in London instead of passing the responsibility to the next parish; and nurturing the physical, mental and moral health of his patients. He preferred prevention to cure, whether of illness or crime and published several novel ideas. They included an early version of the burglar alarm connected to the police station. Blizard proposed hanging a bell in every house, connected by ropes which could be laid along streets in lead pipes. Any break-in could be quickly signalled through these 'reciprocals'.

Sir William was clearly a colourful character. He was one of the last surgeons to consult in a coffee house in the City, a practice common for men of many professions in the eighteenth century capital.[1] He became Royal Surgeon to the Duke and Duchess of Gloucester. As President of the Royal College of Surgeons, he was required to receive the bodies of executed criminals for anatomical dissection – whilst wearing full court dress. Aged 91, he was operated on for cataract and celebrated a successful outcome with one of his numerous poems:

> *The mind invokes, and lights reflective way*
> *To visual sense will forms defin'd decay*
> *The sight, in contemplation's proper scope,*
> *Advances Science, strengthens Christian hope,*
> *All Nature spreads her charms to ravish sight.*

William Blizard died aged 93 and was buried initially at Brixton before his grave was moved to Norwood where it remains to this day.

The Blizard Building is on the Whitechapel campus

---

1   Wags are fond of saying that Lloyds of London began in a Coffee House and landed up in a percolator, a reference to the Rogers' building.

Henry Edmund Gaskin Boyle
1875-1941

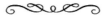

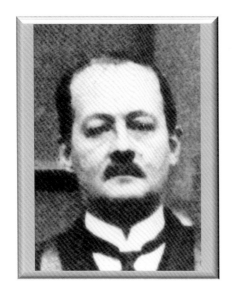

Henry Boyle is the father of English anaesthetics. The equipment he developed for the storage and delivery of gaseous anaesthesia became the prototype for machines in use today; older anaesthetists still refer to 'Boyle's machine' and the 'Boyle's Bottle'. During World War One, he worked with the Royal Army Medical Corps, publishing the results of over 3,600 cases, and was awarded the OBE. He was a founding member of the Journal of Anaesthetists and was the President of the Section of Anaesthetists of the Royal Society of Medicine.

Henry Boyle was born in Barbados, the only son of estate manager Henry Eudolphus Boyle with his wife Elizabeth and was educated at Harrison College, Bridgetown. He came to England in 1894 and entered Barts as a medical student, qualifying in 1901. After a year in Bristol, he returned to Barts as a junior anaesthetist and was appointed consultant in 1903.

By 1900, anaesthesia was moving forwards. The 'rag and bottle' technique of delivering chloroform, famously employed by Dr. John Snow for the delivery of Queen Victoria's last two children, Leopold and Beatrice, risked dangerous side effects. Anaesthetic agent was dripped from a bottle onto a lint cloth over the patient's face, but despite a frequent removal of the lint, chloroform was hepatotoxic and ether could cause pulmonary complications.

In order to use nitrous oxide, the preferred new and safer anaesthetic option, Henry Boyle designed a heavy wooden box with four cylinders hung from metal crossbars. Above them were the vapouriser and the ether container, attached by tubing to a respiratory bag and mask. Boyle was left-handed and the various taps, flow meters and bubble chambers were arranged for his convenience and remain so today! To overcome the problem of a gas freezing up, his first machine contained a spirit lamp whose open flame warmed the reducing valve, dangerously close to highly combustible ether. Through the 1920s and 1930s, Henry Boyle improved his machine, introducing bypass controls, warm water jackets and pressure-reducing regulators, modern forms of which are still in use.

Henry Boyle travelled extensively in North America and shared his ideas with fellow anaesthetists. He met James Gwathmey, now First President of the American Association of Anaesthetists, in New York and attended the first meeting of the Canadian Society of Anaesthetists in Ontario. He brought back the Davis gag for dissection tonsillectomy, a modified version of which is still in use.

By all accounts, he was a stimulating lecturer: most of his teaching was practical and carried out in the operating theatre. He trained many of the early 20th century anaesthetists, perhaps responsible for the tradition, 'you could always trust a Barts man to give a decent anaesthetic'. (Women were not appointed anaesthetists at Barts until after the second World War.)

He died in October, 1941.

The Boyle Room is on the West Smithfield campus

Sir Robin Brook

1908 - 1998

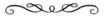

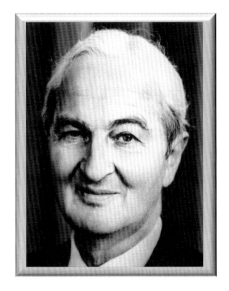

Robin Brook became the first Chairman of the Board of Trustees, set up in 1974 to administer endowment funds for Barts, a role to which he gave unique authority and wisdom and in which he continued until his retirement in 1988. He remained as informal investment advisor until his death in 1998. Previously, Sir Robin had been Chairman of the Barts Board of Governors from 1969, bringing together interests in medical charities and finance in the City of London. It was Sir Robin as Chairman who accompanied the Queen when she attended Barts 850th anniversary celebration in 1973.

Brook recognised the need for the Barts Trustees to play a wider role if the hospital was to respond to changing pressures in the NHS: major contributions built new operating theatres and funded expensive equipment, including the first CT scanners. In the late 1970s, when research was expanding and space was limited, Sir Robin led an appeal for funds which led to the establishment of the Barts Research Development Trust, which he chaired until the 1990s and which provided an extra 35,000 square feet of available space. Brook's Trustees contributed substantially to the Medical Education Centre, 1980, a development which bears his name and which revolutionised undergraduate and postgraduate teaching at Barts. He became President and Chairman of the Council of Barts Medical College, a post he held for nearly twenty years.

Robin Brook was born in 1908, the son of a surgeon, and was educated at Eton and Kings College, Cambridge. He was awarded a Double First in

Economics, studying under Maynard Keynes, and finding time to fence for the University, later representing Great Britain in the 1936 Olympics and again postwar in 1948. He became a Special Operations Executive in the second World War, an undercover organisation that helped resistance movements in enemy-occupied territory. Brook not only recruited agents, but also took part in Special Operations Executive activities in Western Europe for which he received many honours including the French Legion of Honour and the Belgian Croix de Guerre. He was probably involved in secret pacts between Britain and America to share intelligence and code-breaking operations against Nazi Germany.

In 1945, he was appointed a governor of the newly-nationalised Bank of England – at 37, the youngest ever. His financial skills were much in demand when he served, often as Chairman, on many committees and boards, both in the City and in public service. He was appointed CMG in 1954 and knighted in 1974 for services to industry.

He was married to Helen whose legacy remains the Brook Advisory Centres. Family Planning, pioneering work for sexual health and education for young women, is now taken as standard practice, but it was the subject of fierce opposition in 1963. Robin Brook's support to Helen's initiative cannot be overestimated; he drafted its constitution, established the framework and acted as facilitator and financial advisor.

In the many obituaries that paid tribute to him following his death in December 1998, Sir Robin was described as 'a quiet man, almost diffident, but with a steely core, allied to intelligence, enthusiasm and clarity of thought, which made him an effective leader'. He could appear intimidating but closer acquaintance revealed a stimulating companion with a wicked sense of humour.

The Robin Brook Centre is on the West Smithfield campus

Yvonne Carter
1959 - 2009

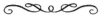

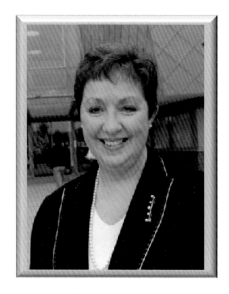

Yvonne Carter became the youngest professor of general practice and primary care in the UK at Barts, newly merged into Barts, the London, and Queen Mary Westfield School of Medicine and Dentistry in 1996. She sought to facilitate higher academic roles for women doctors and was awarded the CBE in 2009 for services to medical education. From a broad and extensive spectrum of published research, she achieved lasting recognition for her studies of palliative care and the knowledge needs of informal caregivers.

Professor Yvonne Carter was born in Liverpool and qualified in medicine at St. Mary's, London in 1983. Her return to Liverpool to support her dying mother was responsible for the introduction to paediatrician Michael Bannon at Alder Hey Hospital, whom she married in 1988. Professor Brian McGuinness, then senior partner at the Runcorn practice in Cheshire where she trained, fostered an interest in General Practice. She credited him with demonstrating the possibility of combining general practice with an academic career and inspiring a love of what she dubbed 'clinical generalism'. Her success in the field led her to become one of the leading lights of research practice and innovation at the Royal College of General Practitioners where she developed, amongst a wide variety of initiatives and publications, a research practice accreditation scheme.

In 1990, she accepted a Research Training Fellowship at Keele before moving to Birmingham in 1992 to become Senior Clinical Lecturer. In 1996, she returned to Barts where she remained for nearly ten years as Professor of General Practice and Primary Care. During her tenure, academic primary care in East London underwent a renaissance – general practice in underprivileged areas was a particular interest and engagement. Her reputation as a clinical academic was founded on combining a basic love of doctoring with a rigorous approach to medical research.

This combination of academic and practical medicine was responsible for her vision of the medical school as an important link between a University and the local community. Her own highly developed professionalism was dedicated to raising standards in medical education, academic research and patient care; she had valued experience in all three and strove to maximise links between them.

Professor Carter remained a working GP for over twenty years. In 1994, she became a Fellow of the Royal College of General Practitioners and was proposed as a Member of the Council from 1994-2004. She was the appointed Dean of the new Warwick Medical School in 2006, one of only three women to hold such a position in the UK, but her health was already failing, and she died of breast cancer in 2009.

The Yvonne Carter Building is on the Whitechapel campus

A.E. Clark-Kennedy
1893 - 1985

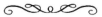

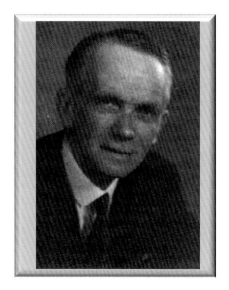

Archibald Edmund Clark-Kennedy, always known as C-K, was Consultant Physician to the London, Dean of the London Hospital Medical College during the Second World War, and Fellow of Corpus Christi College, Cambridge. He was beloved as an eccentric who often rode his horse in Whitechapel, followed hounds, walked the Pennine Way in fourteen days when he was 78 (to become as fit as possible for a cataract operation) and wrote scholarly biographies and medical history. His two-volume History of the London Hospital was completed in 1964.

C-K was born on St. George's Day in 1893 and educated at Wellington College. He followed his father to Corpus Christi where he read Natural Sciences and began a study of medicine at The London. Before he could qualify, the First World War broke out and he saw active service in India and the Middle East. Returning to complete his studies in 1917, he joined the Royal Army Medical Corps and went to France as a medical officer in the Royal Field Artillery.

He rapidly acquired higher medical qualifications, obtaining an MRCP in 1921 and an MD in 1923. He was made a Fellow of Corpus Christi in 1919 and tutored in Natural Sciences. In 1928, he became Physician to the London and an FRCP in 1930. A double life between Cambridge University and London Hospital meant commuting between them by train which C-K used as an office. Railway commuting may be familiar today, as indeed may travelling offices, but neither were standard practice in the 1920s, and the dual responsibilities of University don and London physician remain extremely rare.

C-K's famous energies were put to good use exploring the philosophy of medicine in general and of medical education in particular. He possessed great originality of thought and constantly demonstrated moral courage in demolishing traditional attitudes if they prevented truth; logic was all, common sense was uncommon. In practical terms, C-K was a skilled clinician, teaching that the patient was real and the diseases were an abstraction. This humanism, as he described it in many publications, manifested itself as compassion for the dying and for 'seeing the patient through'. He was an outstanding teacher, lecturing on the proper use of opiates to control pain in terminally ill patients and was one of the first physicians to be defined as a gerontologist. He was an outstanding teacher.

As author, A.E. Kennedy wrote a biography of Nurse Edith Cavell (1865-1915), the humanitarian Stephen Hales (1677-1761) and three stirring accounts of military relations. His medical teaching principles were outlined in a book written near his retirement, *How To Learn Medicine*, Pitman Publishing, 1959.

C-K's long legs and inexhaustible stamina made him a fine sportsman and long distance runner into his 60s and 70s. He continued to ride to hounds when his own eyesight became unreliable, relying on the visual acuity of his horse and after reluctantly abandoning the imbalance of his bicycle, adopted a ten-gear racing tricycle instead. He died in 1985 at the great age of 93 with only a few days of indisposition.

The Clark-Kennedy Lecture Theatre is on the Whitechapel campus

Sir Anthony Michael Dawson
1928 - 1997

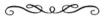

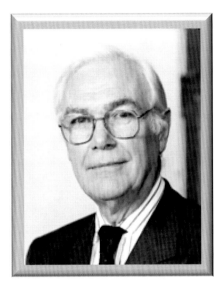

Anthony Dawson was appointed Physician to Barts in 1965 where he practiced with great distinction for over twenty-five years, and remained as Consultant for a further ten. In addition, he was Physician to the King Edward VII Hospital for Officers, 1968-1997, Physician to the Royal Household, 1974-1982, to The Queen, Head of H.M. Medical Household and dubbed a KCVO in 1993. He became a Special Trustee and member of the governing body of St Mary's College during the merger of Barts and the London. Sir Anthony is remembered as both a great physician and an outstanding medical scientist who recognised the profound and indivisible nature of mind and body.

He trained initially at the Charing Cross Medical School, qualifying with honours and the Governor's Clinical Gold Medal. He developed his research interests between 1957-1959 at the Harvard Medical School in Boston where he worked alongside such legendary figures in gastroenterology as Walter Bauer, Chester Jones and Kurt Isselbacher. Tony Dawson's research focused on diseases of the intestine, particularly those which disturbed the absorption of peptides and amino acids through the gut wall. His academic reputation was established with two further years as assistant to Isselbacher at the Massachusetts General Hospital.

Dame Sheila Sherlock, his early teacher and mentor, recognised his distinction and persuaded him to return to the UK and a post at the Royal Free Hospital where she was the first professor of medicine. He became Senior Lecturer before his appointment to Barts in 1965 where his clinical practice expanded to embrace the care of patients with the whole spectrum of gastroenterological disorders rather than any sub-specialism. This breadth of clinical expertise made him much sought after and patients with difficult diagnoses came from all over the UK and beyond, which promoted a highly successful private practice.

His establishment of a position for a psychiatrist within the gastroenterology unit at Barts caused a stir at the time. He was an early scientist to understand and define the relationship of the mind to such disorders as Irritable Bowel Syndrome, and it is no surprise to learn that he was instrumental in setting up a working party with the Royal College of Psychiatrists on the psychological aspects of physical disease, producing a groundbreaking report in 1995.

Anthony Dawson's sympathies extended beyond Barts. He was acutely conscious of social inequalities and difficult access to health care created by homelessness. To this end, he set up a Royal College of Physicians working party, an interest he managed to pursue whilst Vice Chairman of the management board of the Kings Fund,1983-93. He was Chairman of the Council of the British Heart Foundation and Vice Chairman, later Chairman of the Royal Medical Benevolent Fund.

Personally, Tony Dawson possessed a unique blend of intellectual rigour and enthusiasm for everything in life and almost everyone. He was loved for his dedication to his patients and their families and his unfailing sense of humour. Many have cause to be grateful for his interest in good food and wine and a consequent improvement in the College wine cellar. He adored opera, dining with friends at the Garrick and gardening at his home in Culworth. He died a few months before his 70th birthday of a sudden and unexpected heart attack.

The Sir Anthony Dawson Hall is on the Charterhouse Square campus

Israel Doniach

1911 - 2001

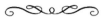

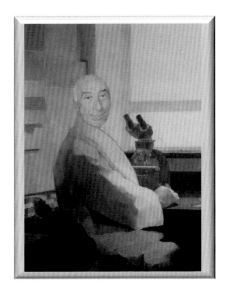

Israel Doniach became a Barts man late in his profoundly distinguished medical career. When he joined St. Bartholomew's, he was sixty-four and had recently retired as Emeritus Professor of Morbid Anatomy at the London Hospital Medical School, known nationwide for his work on the causes and treatments of thyroid cancers. He joined Professor Mike Besser's histopathology research team in 1975 where his practical expertise and wise counsel were to make a considerable contribution to the endocrine world over the next fifteen years.

Israel Sonny Doniach was the son of Russian Jewish immigrants who fled to the East End of London to escape Tsarist pogroms in the early twentieth century. His father, Aaron, was an Arabic and Hebrew scholar who founded the first chair of modern Hebrew at what became the London University School of Oriental Studies; his brother became a code-breaker at Bletchley Park; and his sister was a concert pianist and composer. Sonny studied medicine at University College and graduated in 1934. He studied pathology at St. Mary's Hospital where he published his first work on the interaction of light and carcinogens in nature.

In the early 1960s, Sonny and his colleagues realised the carcinogenic potential of radioiodine for the thyroid gland. He was Reader in Morbid Anatomy at the time and his research was of particular significance as radioiodine was extensively used for the diagnosis and treatment of thyroid disorders. Many years later, this finding was confirmed from the high incidence of thyroid cancer seen in children after the Chernobyl disaster at which considerable quantities of I/131 were released. Doniach and Howard Pelc developed a technique known as autoradiography which permitted localisation of isotope uptake to individual cells. Doniach's autoradiography became a crucial tool for studying cell division – in particular, the role of stem cells in the organisation of other tissues.

Sonny Doniach was a man of gentle, kindly appearance who loved a joke. He delighted in family anecdotes and stories, often told with scurrilous wit. In the 1940s he married Deborah, an outstanding clinical immunologist and authority on auto-immunity who worked at the Middlesex Hospital in London, and one of Sonny's pleasures in life was discussing science with her. Their son Sebastian is professor of physics at Stanford University, USA.

The Doniach Gallery is on the Whitechapel campus

John Langdon Down
1828 - 1896

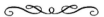

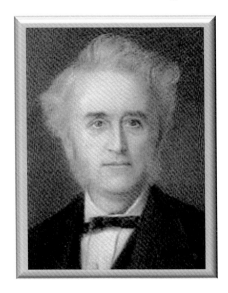

John Langdon Down was a pioneer in the diagnosis and care of those born with the congenital abnormality which now bears his name. Before his work, such mentally handicapped people were commonly described as idiots or mongols and confined in lunatic asylums where their lives amongst the seriously insane were often unimaginably brutal and harsh. He devoted his medical life to helping those he described as feeble in mind; his training systems were based on physical exercise, sensory stimulation and role play. He encouraged and taught carers who would now be classified as speech therapists and special needs teachers.

John Langdon Down was born in 1828 above his father's grocery shop in Torpoint, Cornwall. He left school at 14 and helped in the shop for four years. Aged 18, he was brought into contact with a "feeble minded girl who waited on our party and for whom the question haunted me - could nothing for her be done"? This momentous meeting proved the inspiration for his entire medical career, first as an apprentice to a surgeon in the East End of London and later as a student at the Royal Pharmaceutical Society. Passing his exams, he returned briefly to his father's shop where he developed a successful line of over-the-counter products, but he later came back to the Royal Pharmaceutical Society as a laboratory assistant. Ill health, probably tuberculosis, obliged his return yet again to Cornwall for recuperation where he remained until 1853.

When his father died, John Langdon Down was able to enter the London Hospital Medical School where he won Best Student medal in his final year. He was appointed Assistant Physician and presented a number of papers to the Medical Society of London, including the description of the Mongolian group which led to the specific recognition of this disability as a distinct category. Down defined the characteristic obliquely placed eyes and narrowed palpebral fissue with widened epicanthic folds. He appreciated that the disability was congenital and not secondary to birth trauma. It took ten years for his work and compassion to be recognised and still longer for the term mongol to be replaced by 'Down's Syndrome'. His son, Reginald, recognised the palmer abnormalities.

Langdon Down became Medical Superintendent of Earlswood Asylum for Idiots which sounds pejorative today, but was a step forward in 1855. It was financed entirely by public subscription and housed individuals with all types of mental disabilities, with the specific purpose of educating those with learning difficulties. Patients slept in dormitories of fifteen, and there was one member of staff to every seven inmates. Manual trades such as carpentry and printing were taught, as well as domestic and farm duties. The Asylum was absorbed into the NHS in 1958 and closed in 1977 as part of the plan to absorb people with learning difficulties into the community.

John Langdon Down was a progressive and liberal doctor who was prepared to accept change in many areas of medicine and of life. He promoted the advancement of women in the law and the church, and his Harley Street rooms were a base for the Suffragette Movement.

John Langdon Down House is on the Charterhouse Square campus

Michael Anthony Floyer
1920 - 2000

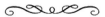

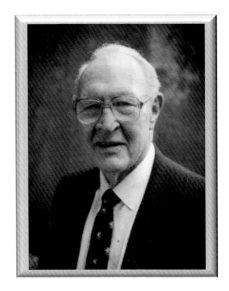

Professor Floyer was Dean of the London Medical School from 1982-1986 and became an early supporter for merging the London Medical Schools. He believed passionately that students should have the benefits of a multi-faculty institute and began preparations for joining forces with Barts in the 1980s. Much of his professional time and energy was directed towards achieving this end. The full merger took place in 1995 and, although it seems obvious with hindsight, it was bitterly contested at the time. Only a few brave and farsighted medical practitioners offered unqualified support.

Mike Floyer was educated at Cambridge and graduated in medicine from the London Hospital Medical School in 1944. His first paper in The Lancet, written in 1946, dealt with the effect of stress in the gut. He measured stomach contents of free hydrochloric acid, total acidity, starch and bile in a group of volunteer medical students waiting for the results of their final examinations. He found that there was no evidence of hypersecretion as stress levels rose and fell before and after the results were announced. 12 students passed and 4 failed their examinations.

After National Service with the Royal Air Force, he was appointed a clinical lecturer on the London Academic medical unit in 1948. His research moved to the role of the kidney in hypertension, and he thought nothing of using himself as an experimental subject. He had a subcutaneous capsule inserted which accumulated interstitial fluids, the composition of which could be measured and studied under a variety of physiological circumstances. In 1980, he was awarded the Oliver-Sharpey Prize at the Royal College of Physicians for his work on hypertension.

In addition to research, Mike Floyer was an enthusiastic teacher. He believed that medicine was a life-long learning experience and that disease should be understood in terms of disorder of structure and function. In addition to his academic duties, Floyer was not only Director of the Accident and Emergency Department but also a general physician with a busy diabetic clinic. In the 1970s, he spent three years as visiting professor at the University of Nairobi where he helped develop the medical faculty. During that time, he was personal physician to Jomo Kenyatta, first President of an independent Kenya.

Out of the wards, Mike Floyer was a keen rugby player and became President of the Royal London Hospital Rugby Team. His contribution is recognised today by the Mike Floyer Memorial Day Match, an annual fixture between current students and Old Boys.

Floyer House is on the Whitechapel campus

Sir Archibald Garrod

1857 - 1936

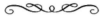

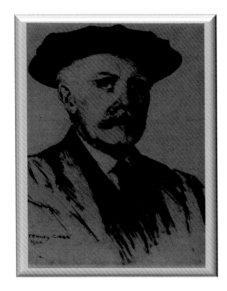

Archibald Garrod was the son of famous Harley Street physician and rheumatologist Sir Alfred Baring Garrod. His father believed he was best suited to business, but his teachers at Marlborough realised that the boy had a penchant for science. He won a first class degree in Natural Sciences from Christ Church, Oxford and, after a short period in Vienna, joined the staff at Barts, becoming first Casualty Physician in 1888 and Assistant Physician in 1903. He developed a particular interest in the inborn metabolic errors which lead to disease and presented his first substantial paper on the topic to the Royal College of Physicians in 1908; this laid the formulation of the crucially important 'one gene, one protein' concept. Although his work was slow to attract the notice of scientific colleagues, it became clear that Garrod had pioneered a new field of medicine.

An undergraduate interest in astronomy had introduced him to Herschel's studies of the nebulae using spectrometry. This led to his appreciation of spectrometry in analysing the composition of gases and other substances, prompting a speciality in chemical pathology as well as more general medicine. By 1908, he had investigated a number of rare, inherited diseases (via autosomal recessive genes) by analysis of the patient's urine. Most notably was alcaptonuria – a condition in which excessive homogentisic acid causes damage to cartilage and to heart valves as well as precipitating kidney stones.

His work was interrupted by the first World War where he served as Consulting Physician to the Mediterranean Forces in Malta. He was awarded a CMG in 1916 and knighted in 1919 for distinguished service to medicine in war. He lost two of his three sons in action and the third died of influenza during the pandemic of 1919. These tragedies profoundly affected Garrod who became more of a laboratory man, avoiding the wards where possible, but never losing sight of clinical medicine.

On his return from wartime duties in 1919, he became director of a new medical unit at Barts, but less than a year later, he was appointed Regius Professor Medicine in Oxford. Garrod's formal style and reserved manner as chemical pathologist and doctor were in considerable contrast to those of his predecessor, the teacher and physician of bedside medicine, Sir William Osler.

Garrod's final treatise on Inborn Errors of Metabolism, 1923, which mostly dealt with rare illnesses that physicians seldom saw (cystinura and pentosuria, for example) was still ahead of its time; it took another ten years before 'biochemical individuality' was recognised.

Sir Archibald was a founder of the Association of Physicians and received honorary degrees from the Universities of Aberdeen, Dublin, Glasgow, Malta and Padua. He was a Fellow of the Royal Society and Vice President from 1926-1928. In 1935, he was awarded the Gold Medal of the Royal Society of Medicine. Contemporaries described him as a quiet and courteous man of rare charm, universally respected and liked, but too gentle and honest to demand attention.

The Garrod Building is on the Whitechapel campus

William Harvey
1578 - 1657

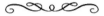

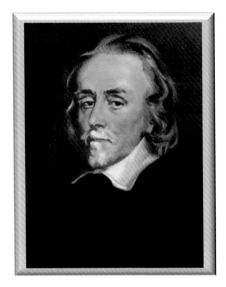

William Harvey, a Barts man for thirty-five years, was the first English physician to discover the circulation of the blood. For more than 1400 years, it was believed that the blood moved to and fro in the vessels, contained air, and passed through pores in the septum of the heart that separated the two ventricles. An Arab polymath, Ibn al-Nafis, doubted this Greek pulsation theory and suggested pulmonary circulation, but this was not believed in 17th century Europe. It was not until the meticulous observation, experiments and research by Harvey, probably in his own house on Ludgate Hill and presented to College of Physicians, that his circulation theories began to be accepted and understood.

William Harvey was born in Folkstone on April 1st, 1578 and educated at King's, Canterbury. He won a scholarship to Cambridge to study medicine and graduated in 1597. Severe ill health, probably malaria, endemic in the fens at that time, prostrated him for two years, but he recovered sufficiently to continue his studies in Padua. Under the guidance of Fabricius, one of the great Italian anatomists, he began his concentration on the vascular system and received his doctorate in 1602.

He was accepted into the College of Physicians on his return to England and was supported by James I in his application to Barts during 1609. His duties were to attend at least one day a week in the Great Hall, to see and prescribe for patients and to visit at the request of Matron. He became friend and adviser to Charles I and was lucky not to be persecuted as a Royalist after the Civil War.

Harvey's laboratory books were destroyed during the Cromwellian parliament, probably because of his association with royalty. But surviving publications prove his discoveries; the valves in the heart direct blood to the pulmonary artery from the right, the aorta from the left and the septum is not porous. He showed that the movement of blood in the veins is always towards the heart, not away from it, postulating that some unseen network existed between the arteries and the veins. (Microscopes needed to observe the capillary network were not perfected until later in the 17th C.)

Professor Dame Lesley Rees inaugurated William Harvey Day during her Deanship of St. Bartholomew's Medical College and this is now held annually on the day nearest Harvey's first admission to Barts. Distinguished speakers from all over the world arrive for presentations, a commemoration service at St. Bartholomew The Great and a subscription dinner at the Museum of London.

The William Harvey Research Institute is on the Charterhouse Square campus

Richard Michael Mason
1917 - 1977

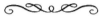

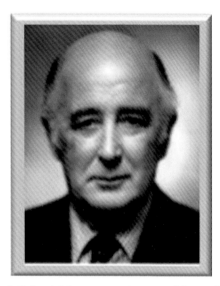

Richard Michael Mason, always known as Michael, was a pioneering rheumatologist. He collaborated closely with surgeons for early treatment of rheumatoid arthritis in contrast to using it as a last resort. His example has been widely adopted and is now routine. As co-editor, he produced the standard rheumatology text book *Mason and Currey* and contributed chapters to many medical reference books, journals and scientific papers.

Michael Mason was born and brought up in India. He was educated at Marlborough College and Oxford University before service with the Royal Air Force during World War II. He entered St. Bartholomew's Medical College and became a Registrar, narrowly missing an early death during the Blitz when a bomb fell on his bedroom floor – he was on the wards at the time. Mason began to specialise in rheumatology and trained with Dr. W.S. Copeman at the West London Hospital, achieving status as Consultant Rheumatologist at the London in 1955. The department to which he was appointed was called Physical Medicine but he transformed it into one of the most influential centres for rheumatoid disease in the country. As Chairman of the Arthritis and Rheumatic Council, he was responsible for building laboratories for research into rheumatic diseases at the London, one of which became the Michael Mason room.

Among his research interests were clinical drug trials, polymyalgia rheumatica and sero-negative arthritis. He was a fine diagnostician and a master at eliciting physical signs and symptoms. Out of the wards, he was an efficient fund-raiser for research and greatly increased the income of the

ARC during his tenure as Chairman. Michael Mason was equally skilful as a mediator and deftly led the negotiations which laid the foundations for accreditations and further rheumatological developments.

In 1967, he travelled to Australia as visiting Professor to Sydney University. This inspired an Australian Rheumatic Association which set up a fellowship to encourage the exchange of junior staff between the UK and Australasia.

Michael Mason was President of the British Association of Physical Medicine and Rheumatology, the Heberdon Society and the British League Against Rheumatism. There is an annual Fellowship in his name to encourage excellence among the younger members of the British Society of Rheumatology.

In private life, Michael was a devoted family man, a keen skier and an expert sailor. His wife Heather was constantly on standby with suitcases packed and meals cooked as sustenance for either tireless professional duties or energetically recreational forays. He died of a sudden heart attack during the XIV International Congress of Rheumatology, a few weeks before his planned retirement.

The Michael Mason Room is on the Whitechapel campus

Sir Michael Willcox Perrin
1905 - 1988

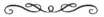

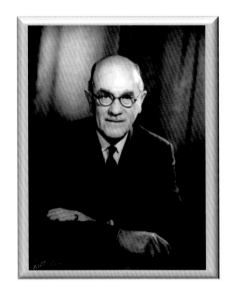

Michael Perrin's immensely distinguished career combined science, charitable finance and administration. At the forefront of polyethylene development, he was also involved in atomic science and nuclear research. His public service appointments included becoming Treasurer and then President of the Barts Medical College before his tenure as Chairman of the Governors of Barts from 1960-1969.

Michael Perrin's father was Bishop of Columbia and he was born in Victoria, British Columbia, in 1905. The family moved to England in 1911 where Michael attended Winchester College before going up to New College, Oxford, to read Chemistry. After graduating, he qualified further with a physics degree from the University of Toronto. Perrin returned to England and joined Imperial Chemical Industries where he led a team investigating polymerisation which patented the first practical method of producing polythene.

As so often, it was a happy accident which produced the milky substance derived from petroleum, even if its practical use was initially unclear.

At the outset of World War II, Perrin had become Assistant Research Director of ICI and was seconded to a committee to advise the government on building an atomic bomb. (He helped the Danish Nobel Prize winning physicist Niels Bohr to escape Nazi persecution.) During the war, Perrin's team worked on atomic science in secret in the UK but his suggestion that it would be better to cooperate with the Americans was accepted and he became British Government Coordinator of the Manhattan Project.

His position made it possible for him to gain covert information on the German atomic programme and he played a major part in disrupting it. Later, he wrote the story of Britain's role in developing the atomic bomb.

Postwar, Michael Perrin was appointed Deputy Controller of the Atomic Energy Authority, 1946-1951, and he supervised the use of nuclear power for peaceful as well as military purposes. He left public service in 1951 and returned briefly to ICI before his appointment as Chairman of the Wellcome Foundation, the commercial outcome of Sir Henry Wellcome's legacy, wholly owned by the charitable Wellcome Trust. Perrin used the profits of the Foundation to expand the business into one of the biggest and most successful drug companies in the world. When he retired in 1970 the Trust had become one of the world's wealthiest charities and Barts became one of its many beneficiaries. Michael Perrin was made an Honorary Perpetual Student of Barts Medical College, an honour accorded mostly to distinguished visiting physicians, but exception was made for a man whose gifts benefited the hospital with so much scientific and financial expertise.

Three bishops attended the wedding of Michael Perrin to Nancy Curzon: his father, then Bishop of Willesden; her father, the Bishop of Stepney; and the Bishop of London, who gave the address. They had a son and daughter and lived all their lives in Hampstead where Michael died in 1988 at the age of 83.

The Perrin Lecture Theatre is on the Whitechapel campus

Dame Lesley Howard Rees
1942

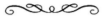

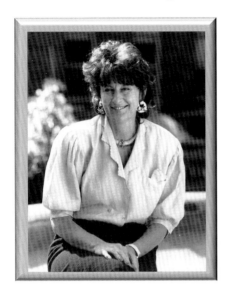

Lesley Rees became the first woman to be appointed sub-dean at Barts Medical College and then the first woman to become Dean in 1987. She had begun her medical career at the age of only seventeen at Barts, a hospital to which she devoted her entire professional life and in which she achieved international recognition for her research and practice in endocrinology. In a continuing series of firsts, she became Professor of Chemical Endocrinology in 1978, the youngest woman to be appointed to a London University Chair in medical science.

Lesley was born in Aberdeen during World War II. Her early life was marred by family tragedy; her father, Flying Officer Howard Davis, was killed in action before her birth and her mother died in a car crash when Lesley was sixteen. Tenacity and courage got her through education at Pates Grammar School and Malvern Girls College before she arrived at the masculine-dominated world of Barts in 1960.

Lesley Rees made her mark early in the Medical College as a charismatic doctor with a unique personal touch and a flair for fashion. Professor Michael Besser recruited her to his pioneer Endocrinology Unit and, together with John Landon, they created a research department to rival any in the world. In the 1970s the team discovered a group of neuro-peptides (that we now call 'endorphins') in the brains of animals. Rees and her colleagues were able to demonstrate the presence of these peptides in human life and to elucidate their structure and function. Her research included proving the actual scientific basis for acupuncture in the relief of chronic pain.

In 1987, as Dean, Lesley was given the task of reforming medical education at Barts. Not only was the old apprentice model rapidly becoming out of date, but advances in medical science made the curriculum unmanageable in its existing form. Moreover, Government Reports on Health and Hospitals in London were proliferating, to no effect whatever, although all concerned realised that the London-centric basis was inefficient and unfair. Lesley initiated the first Clinical Skills Laboratory over the Robin Brook Centre which aimed to teach self-directed learning through independence and discovery. In this process, students would appreciate that they are dealing with people, patients and disease, not abstract scientific phenomena. Lesley Rees was also responsible for a new collaboration with the College of Nursing.

Eventually, the Tomlinson Report achieved what earlier studies had not managed to do, threatening the very existence of Barts in the process. A huge public outcry saved the Medical College from extinction, but could not guarantee its independence, and a merger between Queen Mary Westfield, the London School of Medicine and Dentistry and Barts Medical College was achieved in 1995. Lesley retired as Dean to become Director of Education at the Royal College of Physicians and took charge of the International Office.

Since then, she has served with numerous medical charities including the Winston Churchill Memorial Trust, the Jean Shanks Foundation and Breakthrough Breast Cancer, responsible for introducing the Prince of Wales as Patron. Lesley Rees co-authored *Medical Education in the Millenium* for Oxford University Press in 1998 with Brian Jolly and continues an active involvement with Barts, notably with Professor Gerald Libby's campaign to save the fabric of the Great Hall. Her unique contribution to medical education was rewarded with a DBE in 2001.

In 1969, Lesley married Gareth Rees who became Senior Cardiothoracic Surgeon at Barts. They live in Hampstead with frequent forays to fish in Herefordshire and visits to their French cottage on the Isle de Re.

Dean Rees House is on the Charterhouse Square campus

Sir James Paterson Ross
1895 - 1980

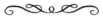

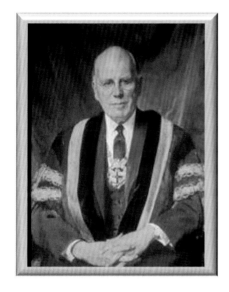

When medical schools in the capital became affiliated with London University, new professorial units were established in Medicine and Surgery. James Ross became the second Professor of Surgery at Barts in 1935, succeeding Professor George Gask for whom he had become an Assistant in 1923. He is remembered at Barts for firmly establishing the Surgical Professorial Unit at the centre of medical education and research, using the expertise of pathologists, radiologists and radiotherapists, as well as consulting specialist physicians in order to obtain and evaluate the best possible treatment for patients.

James Ross was born in London on May 26th, 1895, to an official in the Bank of England. He was educated at Christ's College, Finchley, where he became an outstanding student, winning a science scholarship to Barts and junior scholarships in anatomy and physiology. His medical studies were interrupted by the first World War in which he served as Sergeant Dispenser and, after qualifying on Conjoint, as Surgeon Lieutenant in the Royal Navy.

After the war, Ross trained in neurosurgery in Boston under the American pioneer brain surgeon, Harvey Cushing, a regular visitor to Barts. He returned to work with George Gask in London, researching and practising new surgery on the sympathetic nervous system and the use of radium in the treatment of brain tumours and breast cancer. At the outbreak of World War II, the surgical unit at Barts was evacuated to Hill End, near St. Albans where Ross was in charge of eighty beds. His research at that time necessarily concentrated on war injuries, particularly the bacteriology of wound healing and injuries to blood vessels. In addition, he ran the head injury unit for North London and served on the War Wounds Committee.

When the unit returned to Barts, Ross established a strong research and teaching practice which attained international reputation. In 1949, King George VI developed severe ischaemic symptoms in his leg. He was operated on by Ross and James Learmonth who undertook a lumbar ganglionectomy. Both surgeons were created KCVO and shortly afterwards, Ross attended Sir Winston Churchill to repair a large inguinal hernia with Sir Thomas Dunhill. Anaesthetist Langton Hewer, a Barts man, got a certain pleasure in relating how Dunhill treated Ross as if he were his house surgeon!

James Ross was a shy, selfless man with high ideals. He was liked and admired by students and patients but not universally popular with colleagues who may not have been able to match his humanity and compassion. In 1924, he married Barts ward sister Margaret Townsend. They had three sons, one of whom died in infancy, leaving two remaining boys to become surgeon doctors.

The Paterson Ross Lecture Theatre is on the West Smithfield campus

Sir Joseph Rotblat
1908 - 2005

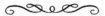

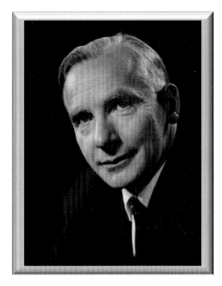

Joseph Rotblat was Professor of Medical Physics at Barts from 1950 to 1976. His long tenure coincided with the increasing dependence of medical technology on physics in general and nuclear physics in particular – Rotblat's speciality. He led a team developing the therapeutic uses of particle accelerators and, in partnership with Patricia Lindop, did extensive work on the effects of radiation on living organisms. He was particularly interested in the consequences of radiation on ageing and fertility and in strontium-90 which alters the composition of bone. He became an international authority on the effects of radiation on human life, travelling extensively all over the world (economy class), lecturing and writing into his ninth decade. Joseph Rotblat wrote over 300 books and papers on medical physics, radiation biology and the hazards and consequences of nuclear war. He was elected FRS in 1995 and knighted in 1998.

Rotblat was born in Warsaw in 1908. His father bred horses in the Polish countryside but their idyllic life changed dramatically at the outset of World War I when the horses were requisitioned for the army and the business collapsed. A wave of anti-Semitism didn't help: thrust into penury, the family was forced to move into a wretched flat with no bath and an outside toilet. The wartime hardship, illness and intolerance that he experienced hardened his resolve to work for world peace. Aged 12, he trained and qualified as an electrician, taking evening classes to win a Master's Degree from the Free University of Warsaw.

At the age of 31, he took up an appointment at Liverpool University and just two days later, Hitler invaded Poland. Joseph Rotblat's wife and mother were taken to a concentration camp where they both died, although Rotblat did not learn of his wife's death for four years. He was seconded to the Manhattan Project, but when he learnt that the American motive for building a nuclear bomb was to use it on Russia, he resigned. From that moment, he worked for the peaceful use of nuclear power. He was a Founder Member of the Campaign for Nuclear Disarmament and Secretary General of the Pugwash Conferences whose mission was 'to bring scientific insights and reason to bear on threats to human security arising from science and technology in general and above all from the catastrophic threat posed to humanity by nuclear and other weapons of mass destruction'.

When he was appointed Professor of Medical Physics at Barts, an initial hostility from certain staff at Barts threatened his arrival and he was forced to delay leaving Liverpool for some months. As a physicist, he was treated as an outsider and his only friend became the Australian endocrinologist A.J.Marshall; neither took kindly to the blimpishness of the then medical establishment. Eventually the doctors, notably Sir Geoffrey Keynes, came to admire and respect him. He was Treasurer of Barts Medical College from 1974-1976.

In 1995, Sir Joseph was awarded the Nobel Peace Prize and he donated the prize money to Pugwash activities. At his death at the age of 97, he was described as '*a towering figure in the struggle for peace; brilliant, eloquent, demanding, impatient and completely committed to the pursuit of a saner, safer world for all of its inhabitants*'.

The Joseph Rotblat Building is on the Charterhouse Square campus

Rev S.A. Thompson-Yates
1843 - 1904

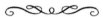

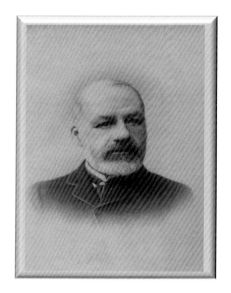

S.A. Thompson-Yates was a philanthropic parson whose charitable donations from his family fortune enabled the building and establishing of medical foundations in Liverpool. His munificence extended to The London where a pathology gallery of specimens is now known as the Teaching Collection in the Thompson-Yates room.

S.A. Thompson-Yates was born in the North of England, the son of G.H. Thompson, a millionaire Liverpool banker in the early years of Queen Victoria. He adopted the extra name Yates from his mother Elizabeth, granddaughter of the Rev. John Yates, and followed his great-grandfather into the Church. Thompson-Yates began his clerical duties as a curate in Lancashire but little is known of his life as a priest.

In the 1850s, Thompson-Yates' Great Uncle, R.V. Yates, had a vision of creating a Medical University College in Princes Park, about a mile south of the existing Liverpool University Campus. This began to take shape in the 1880s and Thompson-Yates offered the unimaginable sum of £15,000 to build a permanent home for both the pathology and the physiology departments. These were completed in 1898. The first Professor of Pathology in the new Thompson-Yates room was Rupert Boyce from University College, London; the first Professor of Physiology was Charles Scott Sherrington, FRS whose work on neuro-physiology won him a Nobel Prize in 1932.

Lord Lister officially opened The Liverpool Thompson-Yates building, unveiling a plaque by local sculptor C.J. Allen. The art nouveau bas-relief depicts allegorical figures of pathology and physiology, believed to have been modelled from the wives of Boyce and Sherrington.

The good Rev. Thompson-Yates devoted his life to medical charity. After the death of his father, he became a man of considerable means and spent his fortune on hospital endowment and his time to giving noble speeches. He pleaded eloquently for greater individualism in national life and less reliance on help from legislation. He urged students not to be satisfied with professional knowledge only but to cultivate in some degree, the study of philosophy, poetry, history and literature. He migrated South and lived in Commercial Road near the London Hospital. He died of kidney failure aged sixty-one.

The Thompson Yates Room is on the Whitechapel campus

Hubert Maitland Turnbull

1875 - 1955

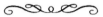

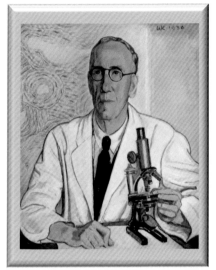

Hubert Turnbull was Professor of Morbid Anatomy at the London for the first half of the twentieth century. When he first entered the practice of pathology, morbid anatomy was considered, literally, a dead subject. Turnbull determined to raise it to the level of a science and he was so successful in this ambition that he inspired not only his colleagues but a generation of young graduates who sought to emulate him.

Maitland Turnbull was born in Glasgow but his family moved to Edinburgh when he was an infant. His maternal grandfather was MP for Edinburgh and twice Lord Provost, with a statue in Princes Gardens. Turnbull received a classical education at Charterhouse School where only one hour a week was allowed for science and even that stopped at the Lower VIth. In consequence, he read Greats at Oxford, obtaining a good second degree. Post-graduation, he was able to study pathology at the new Oxford course for medical students which proved both enjoyable and successful. Turnbull had a good visual memory, passed his 2nd MB and became a demonstrator in anatomy to prepare for his primary FRCS. He thought he wanted to become a surgeon.

In 1902, Turnbull qualified in clinical studies at The London. He was appointed to various house jobs but five months' absence due to serious ill health made him revise his first ambition and he decided that a career in pathology would be more appropriate. He worked in Denmark and Germany where several continental pathologists proved a defining influence.

When he returned to The London in 1906 as Director of the Institute of Pathology, he determined to make radical changes, despite considerable opposition from the old guard. Accuracy of observation and meticulous attention to detail led him, for example, to replace the customary habit of describing tumours as 'pea' or 'orange' size. He emphasised the importance of a variety of staining techniques for microscopical specimens, which led to histochemistry as we know it today. Daily autopsies were conducted for clinicians and students, and visiting pathologists were invited to attend.

His most significant work probably remains post-vaccinal encephalomyelitis. He saw his first case in 1912 and by 1914, he was advising a commission to the Ministry of Health. Turnbull pioneered work on the aetiology of poliomyelitis and made a histological study of encephalitis lethargica, a pyrexia illness that appeared during and briefly after the first World War, but has rarely been reported since.

The relatively few papers he wrote during a long career were of exceptional quality. He co-operated with physicians and surgeons, often adding a pathology paragraph (signed with his initials) but rarely putting his name on the paper. An exception was the collaboration with Dr. Donald Hunter on calcium and phosphorous metabolism and the part played by the parathyroids. Turnbull intended to complete his studies in bone metabolism when he retired, but degenerating health made this impossible.

Maitland Turnbull was elected FRCP in 1929, FRS in 1939 and was awarded an Honorary DSc from Oxford in 1945. He died at age eighty in 1955.

The Turnbull Centre is on the Mile End campus

Sir John Vane

1927 - 2004

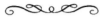

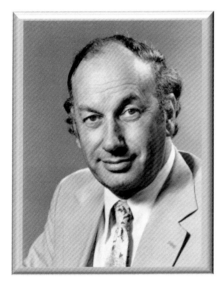

John Vane's pioneering research into aspirin won him a (shared) Nobel Prize for Physiology in 1982. Four years later, he was invited to become a Founding Director of the William Harvey Research Institute at St. Bartholomew's, Charterhouse Square. It became one of the top 20 research institutes in the UK, with a scientific staff of over 130, many of them key researchers in the fields of inflammation and cardiovascular disease. Sir John Vane retired in 1997 and was elected Honorary President of the Institute, retaining friends and a distinguished reputation with Barts.

John Vane was born in Worcestershire and educated at King Edward VI School in Birmingham. He read chemistry at Birmingham University and found the subject boring; he did not expect to find himself persuaded to study pharmacology at Oxford University and had to look up the word in a dictionary. After an Oxford DPhil he became Assistant Professor at Yale University, returning to England in 1955.

Initially, his medical research began at the Institute of Basic Medical Science (next to the Royal College of Surgeons) where he developed bioassay systems. Using small pieces of muscle taken from tissues known to be sensitive to the hormones he was measuring, he was able to measure a number of hormones very accurately in a short time. This led to the ACE inhibitors and treatments for hypertension based on the team's important work on angiotensin.

Vane turned his attention to aspirin. He was able to assay the newly discovered group of chemicals called prostaglandins whose actions caused inflammation, pain and fever. He realised that aspirin might inhibit certain prostaglandins and marshalled the evidence to prove his thesis: he was able to demonstrate that aspirin helped prevent the production of platelets of thromboxane, responsible for platelet stickiness which could cause blood clotting. This explained why aspirin was effective in preventing strokes and heart attacks.

In the 1970s, Vane became Director of the Wellcome Foundation, responsible for the development of anti-viral drugs, and chemical treatments for epilepsy and the prevention of gout. He was elected FRS in 1974.

John Vane was a shy, but sociable man, a good listener and mentor to many young scientists. He attracted the attention of the anti-vivisectionists who carried out a vindictive campaign against him, but he proved an articulate defender of the responsible use of animals in medical research and supported colleagues in the field. He died of pneumonia in 2004, aged 77.

The Sir John Vane Science Centre is on the Charterhouse Square campus

Derek Albert Willoughby
1930 - 2004

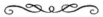

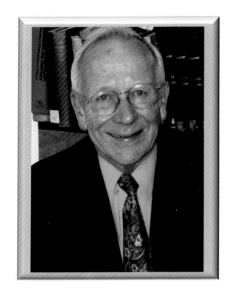

Derek Willoughby became Professor in Experimental Pathology at Barts in 1969 and remained in his post for nearly twenty years. When he retired, he moved to Charterhouse Square as Emeritus Professor where he encouraged John Vane to join the Medical College and to set up the William Harvey Research Institute.

Willoughby was born in North London. His original ambition to become a chef was thwarted by his science teacher at school who convinced his parents that their son should reconsider his career plans. He became a research assistant at University College with Sir Max Rosenheim, producing an assay for phaeochromocytoma which demonstrated a link between that tumour, glycosuria and diabetes. His PhD at Cambridge was a thesis on the role of mediators in irradiation induced injuries, which laid the foundations for further studies on inflammatory mediators and the vascular changes in inflammation. Willoughby's discoveries relating to the inflammatory process have had implications for the treatment of many diseases, but he was particularly interested in patients with rheumatoid arthritis.

He was an outstanding lecturer in the days before white boards and power point, using 35mm slides to great effect. The medical artist Peter Cull drew Willoughby one of the best known illustrations of the inflammatory process and it is still in use today.

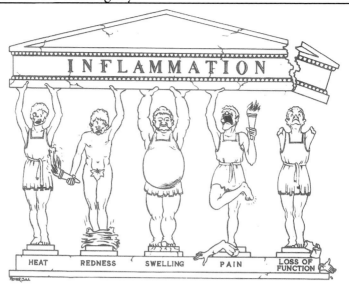

Derek Willoughby wrote as well as he lectured. He produced over 300 original research publications, written in collaboration with the outstanding leaders in the field of pharmacology, pathology and clinical science. He is recognised as one of the outstanding researchers into the science of inflammation in recent years.

Willougby met his wife Pam at University College. He never lost interest in cooking and was known to be an accomplished chef. He was also an athlete, winning medals for 100 and 220 yard sprint, achieving a place in the National Olympic Team.

The Derek Willoughby Lecture Theatre is on the Charterhouse Square campus

David L. Wingate

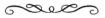

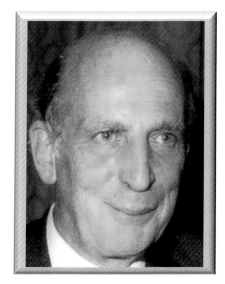

David Wingate became Emeritus Professor of Gastroenterology at Queen Mary College after a distinguished career in gastroenterology at the London. His legacy to medicine remains his work on gut motor activity, whether with interdisciplinary research between gastroenterology, surgery and physiology or with a focus on the neural regulation of motor function and the interaction between the central and enteric nervous system.

Wingate was educated at Oxford University where he carried out research on water absorption in the rat intestine. His resulting thesis was awarded the Gotch Memorial Medal. Post-graduate study at the Middlesex Hospital Medical School included the setting up of his own laboratory, before he moved to the Mayo Clinic to spend a year studying the effects of bile acids on water absorption. He joined the London Hospital Medical College, first as a physiologist and subsequently as a gastroenterologist where his research led to the establishment of a dedicated new unit in 1981. Together with colleagues, he set up a diagnostic centre for detecting gut disorders which has grown into one of the busiest in Europe.

Later studies proved that motor abnormalities of the small bowel can be evoked by stress and are absent during sleep. This produced a popular theory that humans have two brains, one in the gut and the other in the head as well as a new term – neurogastroenterology. (Paleontologists discovered that dinosaurs had two brains; one in the head and one in the tail to speed up a nervous reaction between sensors.)

David Wingate travelled extensively. He was a Founder Member of the European Motility Society and Chairman of the International Motility Symposium in Oxford. In 1989, he and colleagues founded the continuing series of triennal symposia on Brain-Gut Interaction. He served as Joint Editor of the journal Neurogastroenterology and Motility and as Review Editor of Gut.

In 2000, David Wingate retired from his academic post, and the Gastrointestinal Science Research Institute was formally renamed as The Wingate Institute. He remains committed to seeing gastroenterology research activity flourish at the Institute that now bears his name.

The Wingate Institute is on the Whitechapel campus

The Wolfson Family

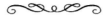

The Wolfson family have magnificently endowed Wolfson colleges and institutes. Health, education, science, the humanities and youth welfare have been the major beneficiaries of their philanthropy in this country for over half a century. In 1959, they gave £450,000 to the Royal College of Physicians and, in partnership with government, have funded projects at the Royal Society, and Museum and Gallery improvements. In 1991, Wolfson was the major donor for the foundation of the Institute of Environmental and Preventive Medicine in Charterhouse Square.

Isaac Wolfson was the son of a Polish immigrant who settled in the rough Gorbals district of Glasgow early in the 20th century. He studied at Queen's Park School in Glasgow where he proved brilliant at mathematics but because he could not afford to train as an accountant, he worked selling the cheap tables and chairs made by his father. In 1926, he was recruited as a buyer for Universal Stores, the leading mail order company for clothing famous for giving credit to its working class customers. Isaac became managing director of Great Universal Stores (GUS) in 1932 and chairman after World War II. By 1955, Wolfson's series of strategic take-overs had built Great Universal Stores into one of the most powerful retailers in the country.

His son Leonard joined him on the board and together they established their Charitable Foundation, initially endowed by six million pounds worth of GUS shares and estimated to be worth some seven hundred and fifty million pounds today. The Wolfsons, father and son, not only shared their orthodox Jewish practice but also belief in philanthropy. Their Foundation has donated in excess of a billion pounds in the promotion of health, education, science, the arts and humanities.

Isaac died in 1991 at the age of 93 and Leonard became Chairman, administering the Wolfson Trust until his own death in 2010 aged 82. Leonard proved to be a shrewd organiser of his philanthropic inheritance. He oversaw the GUS empire which continued to grow until the mid-1990s when stiff opposition from discount stores and cheap credit made inroads into the marketplace. Both father and son were described as enjoying making money and enjoying giving it away.

Leonard Wolfson was passionately interested in history. He appointed historians as trustees of the Foundation and established an annual Wolfson History Prize in 1972 which combined scholarship with accessibility for the general reader. His apartment in Portland Place housed a prize collection of Impressionist and Post-Impressionist paintings of inestimable value.

Isaac was created a baron in 1962 to which Leonard succeeded on Isaac's death. In addition, Leonard was created a life peer as Lord Wolfson of Marylebone in 1985.

The Wolfson Institute of Environmental and Preventive Medicine is on the Charterhouse Square campus